The Miracle of Green Tea

Herbal Remedy for Weight Loss, Diabetes, Blood Pressure, Cholesterol, Cancer, Allergies and Much, Much More

David Sykes

Table of Contents

Introduction

Conclusion

Introduction

I want to thank you and congratulate you for purchasing the book, *"The Miracle of Green Tea"*.

Green tea has been the wonder drink for most people, especially in the Asian region, for years. Ancient physicians and contemporary medical experts have both characterized green tea as a super beverage, as it contains a lot of antioxidants that can cure diseases. Studies show that green tea can actually reduce your risk of cancer and reverse the signs of aging. What this book aims to show you, though, are the other benefits of drinking green tea and why it must be a part of your diet.

This book contains everything you need to know about green tea – from what it is and how it is prepared, to its ancient beginnings, and how science has also proven the effectiveness of the beverage in your health and beauty regimen. It can be a delicious ingredient in your dishes, too.

Keep reading to learn more about green tea and why it is good for you.

Thanks again for purchasing this book. I hope you enjoy it!

This document is geared towards providing exact and reliable information in regards to the topic and issue covered. The publication is sold with the idea that the publisher is not required to render accounting, officially permitted, or otherwise, qualified services. If advice is necessary, legal or professional, a practiced individual in the profession should be ordered.

- From a Declaration of Principles which was accepted and approved equally by a Committee of the American Bar Association and a Committee of Publishers and Associations.

The information provided herein is stated to be truthful and consistent, in that any liability, in terms of inattention or otherwise, by any usage or abuse of any policies, processes, or directions contained within is the solitary and utter responsibility of the recipient reader. Under no circumstances will any legal responsibility or blame be held against the publisher for any reparation, damages, or

Chapter 1 - The Tea as You Know It

In Asia and Europe, locals from the ancient and contemporary times enjoy a cup of green tea. This brew from the *Camellia sinensis* plant originated from China, and was also transported to India and other parts of the world. Even now, green tea is revered as a super drink because of the following benefits:

- Prevents cancer

- Helps regulate cholesterol levels

- Controls blood pressure

- Strengthens the immune system

- Suppresses the growth of tumors

- Reduces the chances of stroke and epilepsy

- Manages blood sugar levels

- Slows down the aging process

It is also astonishing that the Japanese, who drink green tea every day, have longer life spans than most Americans and Europeans. The Japanese's vegan diet helps, but green tea should also be accounted for their good health and long life. In fact, green tea has been considered a medicine in China for 4,000 years and was even called the "divine elixir of the gods". Why wouldn't it be, when it can do a lot of things and its efficacy has been proven by physicians and scientists?

As an evergreen shrub, *Camellia sinensis* grows with fragrant blooms. To reproduce, this plant must be cross-pollinated with another tea plant. They are also not genetically modified; they are grown with care until the leaves are ready for plucking. Even the plucking is done by hands, never by machines, because it could crush or rip off the leaves and results to fermentation – definitely a no-no in the production of tea.

The plucked leaves will then be subjected to processing. They are processed through any of the following means: steaming, withering, drying, rolling, or a combination of these processes. Green tea, specifically, is prepared in these ways: First, it will be steamed after harvesting the leaves. Steaming (some people use the term 'pan-firing') makes the leaves pliable and soft. Next, the leaves will be rolled to lessen the moisture content. The leaves will also be twisted and dried.

The process is done carefully so that the leaves do not lose polyphenols. These are potent health boosters that are present in vegetables and fruits. Their sub-category – catechins – are also powerful antioxidants. To keep the polyphenols in the green tea, the leaves must be pan-fired over charcoal or wood, steamed for about 20-50 seconds, or rotated in heated cylinders for not more than 10 minutes.

Green tea also contains the following:

- Vitamin E that helps slow down aging

- Flavonols that destroy free radicals

- Flouride that prevents the onset of cavities

- Vitamin C that fights stress and infection

- Vitamin B complex that helps in the digestion and metabolism of carbohydrates

Truly, these health promoters make green tea one of the essential beverages in your kitchen. Just imagine loading your system with catechins and these vitamins! You also enjoy the scent of tea, which has a sort of spicy aroma to it. This is why drinking tea is said to have a calming effect – it also caters to all your senses.

Chapter 2 - The History of Green Tea

According to Chinese history, green tea was created when Shen-Nung, a Chinese emperor, was boiling a pot of water and tea leaves flew and dropped to his brew. The tea leaves were then boiled and became what is now known as green tea. Another legend postulates that a Zen Buddhism practitioner traveled to China and meditated by sitting in front of a wall for almost a decade. To keep himself from falling asleep, he cut off his eyelids and these became a tea plant when they touched the ground.

No matter which legend you'd prefer, the most accurate account is that green tea originated from aboriginal natives who lived in Southeast Asia. According to historians, these natives brewed the tea leaves and then drank them. In Burma, on the other hand, tea leaves were not drank but eaten as a salad. The locals of Tibet, in contrast, green tea is mixed with salt, barley meal, and goat's milk butter.

As per historical records from China, Kuo Puo wrote about how green tea was prepared in 350 B.C. Green tea also became popular in China very quickly because of its medicinal properties and as the preferred beverage of the nobility. By 5th century A.D. green tea was drunk for pleasure and a lot of farmers cultivated and harvested green tea plants. This, aside from promoting green tea through word of mouth.

Green tea first reached the West when the Turkish traders bartered with the Chinese. The Turks, in turn, bartered tea with other foreigners, and in 780, tea trading had become so well-known that China had to levy a tax on it. Coincidentally, a Chinese poet named Lu Yu wrote another account on how to prepare and manufacture green tea. He described everything – from the tea plant's origins, to production and cultivation, harvest, drinking, and serving. In short, Lu Yu's work became the major resource of the ancient Chinese who wanted to know more about green tea.

Tea in Japan and Europe

Green tea arrived in the Land of the Rising Sun in the year 729. The monks thought that the tea kept them awake during their meditative practices and decided to plant green tea shrubs in Japan as well. In 794, tea became part of the royal court when Emperor Kammu insisted that he have his own tea garden.

Eisai, a Japanese monk, promoted the drinking of green tea in 1211. He also described the art of the tea ceremony. The tea's "high status" went on for decades, especially during the 16th century, when fierce and strong warlord Toyotomi Hideyoshi became a fan of tea. By 1559, the Western World had become intrigued with the green tea that emissaries were sent to China to get samples of tea leaves for brewing. The royal court then had a taste of how delicious green tea was, and tea became an everyday beverage for the nobles. In 1657, however, tea was served in public in London.

Thomas Garraway, a businessman, even came up with an ingenious way to advertise a rather strange yet refreshing treatment for Europeans, claiming that:

- Green tea battles headache and other pains.

- It is good for the kidney and ureters.

- It relieves one from breathing difficulties.

- It vanquishes bad dreams and aids memory enhancement.

- It makes the body active and lusty.

During the 17th century, Russia got into the business of trading tea with China. Around 300 camels carried four chests of tea across the Gobi desert for three years before they reached Russian plains. This trade influenced the Russian lifestyle. The Russians even invented the samovar, a gigantic water heater and teapot. They made their tea by boiling one part of the tea leaves, and then adding jam or lemon.

By this time as well, European nations knew the healing and relaxing properties of green tea. However, tea was forgotten as soon as it was embraced by the people. France took to drinking wine after a fleeting period of drinking tea; Germany reverted to beer. As for Spain and Great Britain, tea had become a part of their culture.

Tea in India

In 1823, Robert Bruce received a cup of brew from the natives. When he asked to see the source, he was shown the *Camellia assamica*, a different species. Lieutenant Charlton discovered the same thing and sent samples of the tea plant to the Botanical Gardens in Calcutta. Because the East India Company wanted to grow their own tea plants, they also stole seeds of Camellia sinensis from China and cross-cultured tea plants.

As of 1995, India remains to be the largest tea-producing country. China was bumped into second position. This is because the Chinese grew tea plants on small plots of land and production wasn't cheap. Another reason is that they still preferred to prepare and manufacture tea the old-fashioned way, sans the aid of machines. Lastly, the Chinese didn't really advertise tea because they knew that their people would always want it.

Chapter 3 - Tea and Your Health

Cancer is one of the major causes of death in the United States. The cure is sometimes even worse than the disease, not to mention too costly for the patient. A cancer patient who wishes to survive for a few more months or years would have to be subjected to radiation and chemotherapy, two processes which are harmful for the body, ironically speaking. Surely no one likes to have cancer, but you don't have to despair. There are many ways to combat and prevent the Big C, and drinking green tea is one of them!

Green tea contains polyphenols, powerful antioxidants that are also found in garlic, potatoes, fruits, and vegetables. They not only protect the body from free radicals that destroy the cells, but they also strengthen the immune system. During the initiation stage of cancer, polyphenols help neutralize carcinogens and prevent them from corrupting healthy cells. During the activation stage, however, these antioxidants prevent cancer cells from becoming tumors.

To prove the efficacy of green tea in combating cancer, scientists at the Naylor Dana Institute for Disease Prevention (NY) gave a green tea solution to a group of mice. These rodents were likewise injected with carcinogen. After a series of tests and observations for about ten weeks, the experimental group (the mice who were given green tea) had lung cancer, with 12.2 tumors per mouse. In contrast, the control group, which received the same treatment, got 22.5 lung tumors per mouse. This experiment definitely showed that green tea can reduce tumors, thanks to the epigallocatechin gallate (EGCg)

Green tea catechins also prevent cancer through the following ways:

- They lower the toxicity levels in carcinogenic elements.

- They block free radical cells from entering the body.

- They work with antioxidants in the liver, small intestine, and lungs.

- They interfere with the binding of cancer-causing cells and healthy cells.

- They stop or slow down the activation of tumors.

Another good news is that green tea helps fend off the following cancers:

1. Pancreatic cancer. According to studies, people who drank 2 cups of green tea per day decreased their chances of getting pancreatic cancer. The surveys likewise indicated that the increased consumption of green tea lowers the incidence of cancer forming in the pancreas.

2. Esophageal cancer. Non-smoking, non-alcoholic participants in the survey who drank green tea regularly were found to less likely develop cancer in the esophagus. However, drinking the tea while it's burning hot reduced the catechins' effectiveness.

3. Stomach cancer. A case study in Japan revealed that regular green tea drinkers, especially those who took 10 cups every day, had a decreased risk of gastric cancer.

4. Breast cancer. A meta-analysis released in 2006 suggested that green tea could reduce risks of breast cancer, although this claim has yet to be proven through more tests.

5. Colon cancer. In 1990, a study was published in the Japanese Journal of Cancer Research, stating that drinking green tea cam lower the risk of colon cancer.

6. Liver cancer. This has been proven by the mice experiment, so the habit of drinking about 6 to 8 cups of green tea a day could save a lot of human lives.

7. Prostate cancer. Prostate cancer cells grow slowly when the patient drinks green tea on a regular basis.

What Catechins Do

Catechins decrease the toxicity level in carcinogens. Stomach cancer, for example, is the leading kind of cancer in Japan, no thanks to cured, smoked, and grilled meat served in restaurants. Some of these meat products contain N-nitroso compounds, a major cause of stomach cancer. However, studies show that catechins interfere with the transformation of nitrites into becoming more harmful elements.

Green tea also protected the bacteria from aflatoxin. This is produced by a mold that grows on peanuts and is highly cancerous. In fact, aflatoxin has been linked with liver cancer as well as mental retardation.

Another case study was conducted in Shanghai, China, where 711 people with stomach cancer were matched with 711 controls in the same area. The experimental group, however, drank green tea and had 29% lower risk of stomach cancer.

Catechins also interfere with the binding of cancer-causing substances with healthy cells. Once these cells have been attacked by carcinogens, the healthy cells will begin "taking orders" from the cancer cells. On the other hand, catechins from green tea prevent such things from happening.

The catechins from green tea also act as antioxidants that protect the body from free radicals. Green tea's main fighter is

ECGg, which acts like an umbrella over the lipids and fatty acids in the brain. These fatty acids are susceptible to the effects of free radical perodixation, the process responsible for the aging of the brain. ECGg also figures in making the mind more alert.

When ECGg is combined with potent antioxidants such as Vitamins C and E, the power of catechins becomes more pronounced. Moreover, researchers found out that even green tea alone can combat free radicals better than Vitamins C and E can.

The catechins also work in tandem with other antioxidants. This helps strengthen the body's capillary blood vessels, guard against damage to cell membranes, and reduce the oxidation rate of fats.

In 1992, a study in the Cancer Research Journal confirmed that green tea can power up some enzymes and antioxidants in the body. These enzymes are found in the liver, small intestine, and lungs.

Tumor activation is also slowed down, if not abated, by catechins. Researchers at the Laboratory for Cancer Research at Rutgers University in New Jersey have found that giving green tea to mice dramatically inhibited the formation of tumors in the lungs, despite subjecting the rodents to cancer-causing substances consistently.

Though one can't say that green tea can actually stop cancer cells from spreading and ultimately save a person's life, it can definitely be one form of prevention.

Tea and Heart Disease

In the United States, about 500,000 people die of heart attack every year. Heart disease is a sneaky culprit. Unlike cancer, heart attack can come like a thief in the night – unknowingly and sometimes, there would be no way to stop it. Many factors contribute to heart disease: obesity, high blood cholesterol levels, a sedentary lifestyle, cigarette smoking, high stress levels, and diabetes. The good news, however, is that green tea can help mitigate all these factors. It doesn't mean, though, that you wouldn't develop heart disease; it would still depend on your lifestyle and how you take care of yourself. Green tea, on the other hand, can help you lower your risk of heart attack.

It has already been proven in Japan that the more green tea is consumed, the healthier the person becomes because their cholesterol levels are low. A study of 1,371 men in Yoshimi, Japan found that continuous drinking of green tea was associated with lower triglyceride levels.

Green tea also prevents the platelets to clump together. This sticking together of platelets is very dangerous because once the thrombus attaches to the wall of the artery, it protrudes into the bloodstream and obstructs the blood flow. Blood fats, cholesterol, and cellular debris would then be caught in the thrombus and would slowly form a dam that entirely stops the flow of blood. Green tea, however, inhibits the formation of clots and if they do form, ECGg helps break them down.

Epidemiological studies likewise suggest that green tea prevents stroke. Results show that those who drank green tea (5 cups per day) had less than half the incidence of cerebral hemorrhage and stroke than those who drank less.

Green tea also helps keep blood pressure under control. Also known as hypertension, high blood pressure is one sign of heart disease. This is as dangerous as cancer because too much pressure can cause small cracks to form in your artery walls. Consequently, clots could form in these small cracks and will lead to stroke or heart attack. Your heart would have to work so hard to force the blood through the clogged blood vessels until your heart becomes large and simply gives up.

Normal arteries are wide open, flexible tubes that stretch and relax as the blood surges through. However, the blood pressure will increase if the heart beats faster and harder.

If you're the type who smokes a lot, eats too many cholesterol-rich foods, regularly drinks alcohol, does not exercise, or has a poor diet, then you are a likely candidate for heart disease. Fortunately, you have green tea to rely on. Green tea inhibits ACE and lowers blood pressure, without the harmful effects that come from medicine. Green tea was also found to prolong the life span of people who are prone to stroke and heart attack. 500 mg doses of green tea catechins were given to 37 volunteers with high blood pressure, high serum cholesterol, and high blood sugar. The volunteers drank green tea after eating breakfast and lunch every day. At the end of the study, the volunteers' blood pressure and triglyceride levels were reduced to a significant degree.

Green Tea for Diabetics

Diabetes is a condition wherein there is an excess amount of glucose in the bloodstream. It attacks every part of the body. While glucose is considered as the body's fuel, it also needs the help of the insulin. The insulin acts like a key that "unlocks" a cell so that the glucose could enter it. When the insulin fails to do its job, the sugar will remain "unused" and will leave the cell hungry for glucose. The body pushes more and more glucose into the bloodstream until the blood sugar level rises dramatically, but the sugar does not get into the cells. Instead its high levels ravage the body. The long-term damage can be severe such as amputation, kidney failure, ulcer, blindness, and heart disease. One can die from the complications of diabetes.

But green tea helps alleviate the problem. Green tea polyphenols inhibit amylase, a special enzyme that cuts the strings of glucose molecules. Green tea, however, dulls the enzyme's "cutting power" and renders the amylase useless.

In fact, one cup of green tea inhibits 87% of amylase activity.

Losing Weight with Green Tea

Obesity is one major cause of diabetes and heart disease. An obese person generally has higher blood fat levels, cholesterol levels, and an overworked heart. Overweight people are almost six times more hypertensive than slim people.

In a research conducted at Harvard Medical School, 40% of 115,000 women were found to have risk factors of heart disease mainly because they are overweight. Obesity can also be linked to diabetes because the fat cells are accumulated around the insulin receptor sites make it impossible for insulin to "unlock" the cell and the glucose won't be able to get through. Though green tea is not the only solution for diabetes and obesity, it can help a person become slim. People who are conscious about their diet drink green tea every day because it eases digestion.

Tea as Stress-Reliever

Green tea can also be taken to combat stress, which is the emotional, physical, and mental apprehension coming from the demands of daily life. If not managed, stress can take a toll on your body and could even result to heart disease, cancer, and death.

Though there has yet to be a scientific study on the direct effect of green tea on stress, the brew does have a calming effect on the system. This is why some green tea variants are mint-flavored. Meanwhile, the Japanese are also known for their tea ceremony which, according to them, also lessens tension and anxiety.

Chapter 4 - Tea for the Face?

Green tea has many uses, and one of them is as a concealer for eye bags. Cosmetics do work, but nothing beats natural beauty fixes. It does sound unbelievable, but think of green tea as the "jack of all trades" in food and beverages. It can actually do so many things, and its benefits are not limited to health. Aside from fighting cancer cells, diabetes, and obesity, it can:

1. Combat oral bacteria that cause bad breath and cavities.

2. Inhibit the action of viruses, including flu virus, *Vaccinia*, *Herpes*, and even polio.

3. Fight deadly bacteria especially those that cause pneumonia, cholera, botulism, dysentery, abscesses, and food poisoning.

4. Boost your energy without the nasty effects of caffeine such as palpitations and urinary tract infections.

5. Stimulate the immune system and encourage the body to fight against foreign invaders.

6. Slow down the aging process and give you a healthy glow.

7. Maintain the body's fluid balance.

8. Preserve the freshness of cosmetics and food.

According to a traditional Japanese saying, green tea can make the mouth clean. In laboratory tests, green tea catechins inhibited the production of plaque by bacteria called *Streptococus mutans*. These bacteria act on sugars in the mouth and cause plaque buildup. Other experiments even showed that catechins from green tea destroyed the bacteria.

Japanese children who also drank green tea after lunch had fewer cavities than those kids who didn't drink green tea regularly. The study likewise indicated that the bacteria were inhibited right after five to ten minutes of drinking tea. It can also be surmised that tea catechins from green tea are more powerful cavity fighters than fluoride compounds found in toothpaste. This makes green tea an efficient and effective ingredient in herbal toothpaste. It can even be a mouthwash, too.

Green tea can be also be your number one ally against viruses, because green tea leaves have been found to contain an antiviral agent that fights *Vaccinia* virus, *Herpes simplex*, and flu. Green tea catechins inhibit the influenza virus by preventing it from attacking your healthy cells.

In addition, green tea helps you breathe easier. Some people have the bacteria Staphylococcus aureus in their respiratory systems and these bacteria can be the source of infection. When drugs do not work anymore, it means that the bacteria are already resistant to medicine. If the disease is left untreated it may eventually spread to your other bodily systems. Doctors are hesitant to counter the bacteria with stronger medication because the bacteria, being a strong strain as well, might just resist the drug. However, there is hope for patients; they can inhale a solution with catechins to decrease the infection.

Green Tea for the Face?

Aside from literally putting two green tea bags on your eyes to freshen your look, drinking green tea can also help make you look younger. This comes from the free radicals theory. As the catechins fight the free radicals in your body, your cells become healthier, and this manifests on the outside. You get a certain glow, and your wrinkles and fine lines are diminished. It would also help if you take Vitamins E and C, as these complement the catechins found in green tea.

Because the potency of green tea has been tested time and again, it has been included in most cosmetics and body products. Now you could see soaps, lotions, shampoos, conditioners, facial cleansers, toners, and moisturizers laced with green tea extracts. Some facial masks even combine green tea and cucumber.

Does Green Tea Give You Energy?

The scent of green tea alone is an instant pick-me-up. It invigorates the senses because it smells so refreshing. It can also give you the same effect when you drink it. Green tea is much better to consume if you want an energy boost. As compared to coffee, green tea will not make you palpitate. It won't cause muscle tension and irritability. You would also get a good night's sleep with green tea. Though green tea does have caffeine, it's only a mere 15 mg when brewed for 3 minutes, whereas instant coffee has 65 mg of caffeine. It would take four cups of green tea (the strongest variant) to match the caffeine content of drip coffee.

Green Tea and Its Other Uses

Should you stock a lot of green tea bags in your home, don't worry about them being kept in the cupboard. There are so many ways to use green tea, not just a beverage and an addition to your beauty regimen, but also as the following:

1. It can be a food preservative. Seafood dealers even consider dipping the fish in a mixture of water and green tea extract to keep the products fresher for a longer period of time.

2. It can be a food additive. Some chocolates are preserved, thanks to green tea extract. Because of the many health benefits of green tea, its

extract has been infused to chocolates, candies, and other treats.

3. It can pose as a facial cleanser and as other products. Here some cosmetics that use green tea as an ingredient:

Primal Elements Green Tea and Chamomile Soap

Aubrey Organics Green Tea Facial Cleansing Lotion

Aubrey Organics Green Tea and Ginkgo Daily Moisturizer

Earth Science Beta-Ginseng Age-Protective Anti-Oxidant Eye Gel

Freeman Sugar Cane and Meadowsweet Alpha-Hydroxy Facial Scrub

Jason Natural Cosmetics Tea Time
Anti-Aging Moisturizing Crème

D'Arcy Urban Defense Cream

Beauty Without Cruelty Green Tea
Nourishing Eye Gel

Aubrey Organics Green Tea Herbal
Cream Rinse

Aubrey Organics Green Tea Hair
Treatment Shampoo

Aubrey Organics Green Tea and
Green Clay Rejuvenating Facial Mask

Bulgari Eau Parfumee Extreme

Origins Eye Doctor Eye Cream

Primal Elements Phytosome Nutrient
Infusion

Aubrey Organics Green Tea Hand
and Body Lotion with Evening
Primrose

Green tea can also be an ingredient for
toothpaste, mouthwash, and deodorant.
New deodorants now come with green
tea extract. Aubrey Organics' Green Tea,
Vitamin E, and Calendula Natural
Deodorant is safe for children or adults
with sensitive skin. This product has
green tea that acts as an antioxidant
formula, protecting the skin from
perspiration and neutralizing odor. It
also moisturizes the skin.

Chapter 5 - Your Cup of Tea

Green tea is also a wonderful addition to your recipes. It not only makes your dishes delicious, but it also ascertains your family's health. Its delicate flavor isn't overpowering and it blends well with fruit juices and desserts. Try the following recipes at home and indulge in the wonderful taste of green tea.

Green Tea Lemonade

- 1 can (12 ounces frozen lemonade concentrate, thawed)

- 4 ½ cups prepared green tea

Combine green tea and lemonade concentrate. Refrigerate after mixing well. Serve in sugar-frosted glasses. Garnish with a sprig of mint.

Green Tea Mintade

- 2 bunches of fresh mint

- ¼ cup honey

- ¼ cup lemon juice

- 4 cups prepared green tea

Wash mint and place in a saucepan. Add 1 cup green tea and honey. Bring to a boil and simmer uncovered for about 10 minutes. Chill, then strain mint syrup. Add lemon juice and the remaining green tea to mint syrup. Pour over ice in tall glasses and garnish with lemon slices and mint sprigs.

Green Tea Float

- 1 cup prepared green tea, steaming hot

- 2 scoops vanilla ice cream

- Sprigs of mint

Place ice cream, in a tall glass; pour hot tea over it. Add mint sprig to garnish. Makes 1 serving.

Fruity Iced Green Tea

- 4 cups prepared green tea, chilled
- Ice cubes made from fruit juice
- Fruit kebabs

Place fruit juice ice cubes into tall glasses; pour tea over them. Garnish with fruit kebabs. Makes 4 servings.

Apricot Tea Punch

- 1 quart prepared green tea
- 3 cups apricot nectar
- 2 cups orange juice
- ½ cup lemon juice

- ½ cup granulated sugar

- 1 bottle ginger ale, chilled

- Ice cubes

In a pitcher, combine hot tea, apricot nectar, orange juice, lemon juice, and sugar. Mix well and then refrigerate until chilled. At serving time, combine chilled tea mixture with ginger ale in a large punch bowl. Add ice as needed to keep the punch cool.

Green Tea Party Punch

- 2 cups honey, preferably orange blossom or clover

- 3 cups water

- 1 cup mint leaves

- 1 cup orange juice

- 1 cup lemon juice

- 8 cups prepared green tea

- Block of ice

- Slices of lemon and orange

Combine honey and water in a saucepan and stir over medium heat until dissolved. Bring to a boil, add mint, and simmer for 5 mins. Cool and stir. Combine with orange and lemon juices and green tea. Chill thoroughly. Pour the punch over ice in a punch bowl and garnish it with lemon and orange slices. Makes 24 half-cup servings.

Pineapple Green Tea

- 1 ½ cups water

- ½ cup pineapple juice

- 2 green tea bags

- 2 tbsp firmly packed dark brown sugar

In a small saucepan, bring water and pineapple juice to a boil. Set aside and add tea bags. Put the lid on and steep for around 4 minutes. Remove tea bags; stir in sugar. Makes 2 8-ounce servings.

.

Moroccan Green Tea

- 3 green tea bags
- 1 handful of fresh mint leaves
- 3 cups of boiling water

Place tea bags and mint leaves or extract in a teapot. Add boiling water. Steep for 3 minutes. If fresh mint leaves are used, strain. Makes 3 servings.

Green Tea Ice Cream

- 1 pint vanilla ice cream
- 1 ½ teaspoon Matcha green tea (powder)

Slightly soften ice cream. Add the matcha green tea powder and beat mixture until it's well-blended. Freeze until firm. Makes 4 ½ cup servings.

With these recipes, you may even think of making green tea your business. This well-loved beverage and ingredient will surely keep potential customers coming back.

Conclusion

Thank you again for purchasing this book!

I hope this book was able to help you find the many uses of green tea, whether for health, quick beauty fixes, or in the kitchen.

The next step is to buy green tea at your local grocery store and start brewing your cup to enjoy the benefits of catechins.

Finally, if you enjoyed this book, then I'd like to ask you for a favor, would you be kind enough to leave a review for this book on Amazon? It'd be greatly appreciated!

Thank you and good luck!